My Cat's Medical Records

Cat's Name:

____

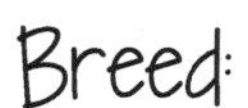

Breed:

Gender:

Birthdate:

Weight:

Length:

Vet's Name:

Vet's Contact Info:

Vaccination Record

Date	Age	Vaccine	Brand	Batch #	Vet

Vaccination Record

Date	Age	Vaccine	Brand	Batch #	Vet

Vaccination Record

Date	Age	Vaccine	Brand	Batch #	Vet

Vaccination Record

Date	Age	Vaccine	Brand	Batch #	Vet

Vet Visit Log

Date Time

Clinic:

Doctor Seen:

Reason For Visit:

Treatment Plan:

Medication:

Vaccinations:

Vet Visit Notes

Vet Visit Log

Date Time

Clinic:

Doctor Seen:

Reason For Visit:

Treatment Plan:

Medication:

Vaccinations:

Vet Visit Notes

Vet Visit Log

Date Time

Clinic:

Doctor Seen:

Reason For Visit:

Treatment Plan:

Medication:

Vaccinations:

Vet Visit Notes

Vet Visit Log

Date Time

Clinic:

Doctor Seen:

Reason For Visit:

Treatment Plan:

Medication:

Vaccinations:

Vet Visit Notes

Vet Visit Log

Date Time

Clinic:

Doctor Seen:

Reason For Visit:

Treatment Plan:

Medication:

Vaccinations:

Vet Visit Notes

Vet Visit Log

Date Time

Clinic:

Doctor Seen:

Reason For Visit:

Treatment Plan:

Medication:

Vaccinations:

Vet Visit Notes

Vet Visit Log

Date Time

Clinic:

Doctor Seen:

Reason For Visit:

Treatment Plan:

Medication:

Vaccinations:

Vet Visit Notes

Vet Visit Log

Date Time

Clinic:

Doctor Seen:

Reason For Visit:

Treatment Plan:

Medication:

Vaccinations:

Vet Visit Notes

Vet Visit Log

Date Time

Clinic:

Doctor Seen:

Reason For Visit:

Treatment Plan:

Medication:

Vaccinations:

Vet Visit Notes

Vet Visit Log

Date Time

Clinic:

Doctor Seen:

Reason For Visit:

Treatment Plan:

Medication:

Vaccinations:

Vet Visit Notes

Vet Visit Log

Date Time

Clinic:

Doctor Seen:

Reason For Visit:

Treatment Plan:

Medication:

Vaccinations:

Vet Visit Notes

Vet Visit Log

Date Time

Clinic:

Doctor Seen:

Reason For Visit:

Treatment Plan:

Medication:

Vaccinations:

Vet Visit Notes

Vet Visit Log

Date Time

Clinic:

Doctor Seen:

Reason For Visit:

Treatment Plan:

Medication:

Vaccinations:

Vet Visit Notes

Vet Visit Log

Date Time

Clinic:

Doctor Seen:

Reason For Visit:

Treatment Plan:

Medication:

Vaccinations:

Vet Visit Notes

Vet Visit Log

Date Time

Clinic:

Doctor Seen:

Reason For Visit:

Treatment Plan:

Medication:

Vaccinations:

Vet Visit Notes

Vet Visit Log

Date Time

Clinic:

Doctor Seen:

Reason For Visit:

Treatment Plan:

Medication:

Vaccinations:

Vet Visit Notes

Vet Visit Log

Date Time

Clinic:

Doctor Seen:

Reason For Visit:

Treatment Plan:

Medication:

Vaccinations:

Vet Visit Notes

Vet Visit Log

Date Time

Clinic:

Doctor Seen:

Reason For Visit:

Treatment Plan:

Medication:

Vaccinations:

Vet Visit Notes

Vet Visit Log

Date Time

Clinic:

Doctor Seen:

Reason For Visit:

Treatment Plan:

Medication:

Vaccinations:

Vet Visit Notes

Vet Visit Log

Date Time

Clinic:

Doctor Seen:

Reason For Visit:

Treatment Plan:

Medication:

Vaccinations:

Vet Visit Notes

Vet Visit Log

Date Time

Clinic:

Doctor Seen:

Reason For Visit:

Treatment Plan:

Medication:

Vaccinations:

Vet Visit Notes

Vet Visit Log

Date Time

Clinic:

Doctor Seen:

Reason For Visit:

Treatment Plan:

Medication:

Vaccinations:

Vet Visit Notes

Vet Visit Log

Date Time

Clinic:

Doctor Seen:

Reason For Visit:

Treatment Plan:

Medication:

Vaccinations:

Vet Visit Notes

Vet Visit Log

Date Time

Clinic:

Doctor Seen:

Reason For Visit:

Treatment Plan:

Medication:

Vaccinations:

Vet Visit Notes

Vet Visit Log

Date Time

Clinic:

Doctor Seen:

Reason For Visit:

Treatment Plan:

Medication:

Vaccinations:

Vet Visit Notes

Vet Visit Log

Date Time

Clinic:

Doctor Seen:

Reason For Visit:

Treatment Plan:

Medication:

Vaccinations:

Vet Visit Notes

Vet Visit Log

Date Time

Clinic:

Doctor Seen:

Reason For Visit:

Treatment Plan:

Medication:

Vaccinations:

Vet Visit Notes

Vet Visit Log

Date Time

Clinic:

Doctor Seen:

Reason For Visit:

Treatment Plan:

Medication:

Vaccinations:

Vet Visit Notes

Vet Visit Log

Date Time

Clinic:

Doctor Seen:

Reason For Visit:

Treatment Plan:

Medication:

Vaccinations:

Vet Visit Notes

Vet Visit Log

Date Time

Clinic:

Doctor Seen:

Reason For Visit:

Treatment Plan:

Medication:

Vaccinations:

Vet Visit Notes

Vet Visit Log

Date Time

Clinic:

Doctor Seen:

Reason For Visit:

Treatment Plan:

Medication:

Vaccinations:

Vet Visit Notes

Vet Visit Log

Date Time

Clinic:

Doctor Seen:

Reason For Visit:

Treatment Plan:

Medication:

Vaccinations:

Vet Visit Notes

Vet Visit Log

Date Time

Clinic:

Doctor Seen:

Reason For Visit:

Treatment Plan:

Medication:

Vaccinations:

Vet Visit Notes

Vet Visit Log

Date Time

Clinic:

Doctor Seen:

Reason For Visit:

Treatment Plan:

Medication:

Vaccinations:

Vet Visit Notes

Vet Visit Log

Date Time

Clinic:

Doctor Seen:

Reason For Visit:

Treatment Plan:

Medication:

Vaccinations:

Vet Visit Notes

Vet Visit Log

Date Time

Clinic:

Doctor Seen:

Reason For Visit:

Treatment Plan:

Medication:

Vaccinations:

Vet Visit Notes

Vet Visit Log

Date Time

Clinic:

Doctor Seen:

Reason For Visit:

Treatment Plan:

Medication:

Vaccinations:

Vet Visit Notes

Vet Visit Log

Date Time

Clinic:

Doctor Seen:

Reason For Visit:

Treatment Plan:

Medication:

Vaccinations:

Vet Visit Notes

Vet Visit Log

Date Time

Clinic:

Doctor Seen:

Reason For Visit:

Treatment Plan:

Medication:

Vaccinations:

Vet Visit Notes

Vet Visit Log

Date Time

Clinic:

Doctor Seen:

Reason For Visit:

Treatment Plan:

Medication:

Vaccinations:

Vet Visit Notes

Vet Visit Log

Date Time

Clinic:

Doctor Seen:

Reason For Visit:

Treatment Plan:

Medication:

Vaccinations:

Vet Visit Notes

Vet Visit Log

Date Time

Clinic:

Doctor Seen:

Reason For Visit:

Treatment Plan:

Medication:

Vaccinations:

Vet Visit Notes

Vet Visit Log

Date Time

Clinic:

Doctor Seen:

Reason For Visit:

Treatment Plan:

Medication:

Vaccinations:

Vet Visit Notes

Vet Visit Log

Date Time

Clinic:

Doctor Seen:

Reason For Visit:

Treatment Plan:

Medication:

Vaccinations:

Vet Visit Notes

Vet Visit Log

Date Time

Clinic:

Doctor Seen:

Reason For Visit:

Treatment Plan:

Medication:

Vaccinations:

Vet Visit Notes

Made in the USA
Coppell, TX
26 May 2022